Top Tips to Prevent and Treat

OBESITY

A novel approach to controlling your weight and health.

COPYRIGHT

TABLE OF CONTENTS

Intentionally left blank

People do get sick occasionally and need pharmaceuticals, but most illnesses cannot be cured by them. Most of the time, drugs don't treat the underlying cause of the sickness; instead, they just help with the symptoms. When the underlying issue is not resolved, it frequently spreads more widely over time. Additionally, using pharmaceuticals to manage symptoms frequently results in the need for more prescriptions, creating a vicious cycle that is contrary to living a healthy life.

Everyone in today's society is searching for the "magic pill" to treat their health issues. We use pills to treat a variety of conditions, including headaches, allergies, backaches, infections, high blood pressure, diabetes, high cholesterol, anxiety, depression, and low energy

SECTION I: THE CAUSE

CAUSES AND PREVENTION OF OBESITY

CHAPTER 1

UNDERSTAND OBESITY

What is Obesity?

Obesity is a long-term condition of the body's weight control mechanisms that are characterized by an accumulation of excess body fat that is significant enough to have a negative impact on health. Genetic, environmental, and psychological elements all contribute to its occurrence. It increases the likelihood of major problems and lowers the quality of life. A pandemic, obesity is a widespread issue that affects a large portion of the world's population. The growth of childhood and adolescent obesity, whose incidence has increased by three times in the past 20 years, is especially concerning.

What are the three types of obesity?

Healthcare providers classify obesity into class types based on how severe it is. They use BMI to do it. If your BMI is between 25.0 and 29.9 kg/m², they put you in the overweight category. There are three general classes of obesity that healthcare providers use to evaluate what treatments may work best for each person. They include:

- **Class I obesity:** BMI 30 to <35 kg/m².
- **Class II obesity:** BMI 35 to <40 kg/m².
- **Class III obesity:** BMI 40+ kg/m².

Nevertheless, Two key hormones play roles in the pathogenesis of Obesity. They are Leptin and Ghrelin.

What is leptin?

Leptin is a hormone your fat tissue (muscle versus fat) delivers that assists your body with keeping up with your typical load on a drawn-out premise. It does this by managing hunger by giving the vibe of satiety (feeling full).

Hormones are synthetic compounds that coordinate various capabilities in your body via helping messages through your blood to your organs, muscles and different tissues. These signs instruct your body and when to do it.

All researchers found leptin in 1994, so they're concentrating on it to see its belongings.

What is the function of leptin?

Leptin's principal function is to assist with controlling the drawn-out balance between your body's food admission and energy use (consumption). Leptin represses (forestalls) hunger and manages energy balance with the goal that your body doesn't set off a craving reaction when it doesn't require energy (calories).

Leptin for the most part follows up on your brainstem and nerve centre to control yearning and energy balance, however, you have leptin receptors in different regions of your body.

Leptin doesn't influence your yearning levels and food consumption from one dinner to another yet rather acts to change food admission and control energy use over a more extended timeframe to assist with keeping up with your typical weight.

Leptin has a more significant impact when you get in shape. As your muscle-to-fat ratio (fat tissue) diminishes, your leptin levels decline, which flags your body to believe that it's destitute. This invigorates deep yearning and craving and can prompt expanded food utilization.

Researchers are as yet considering leptin, and they accept it likewise influences your digestion, endocrine framework guideline and safe framework capability.

How are leptin levels controlled?

Your white fat tissue (muscle-to-fat ratio) makes and delivers leptin. White fat tissue is the fundamental sort of fat in your body. It's situated underneath your skin, around inside organs, in the centre hole of your bones. White fat tissue fills in as padding for different pieces of your body.

How much leptin is in your blood is straightforwardly corresponding to how much fat tissue your body has. All in all, the less muscle versus fat, the less leptin you have, and the more muscle to fat ratio, the more leptin you have.

Leptin levels increment if your fat mass increments over the long run, and they decline your fat mass abatements after some time.

What is ghrelin?

Ghrelin is a hormone produced by your stomach. Other parts of your body, such as your brain, small intestine and pancreas, also release small amounts of ghrelin.

Often known as the "hunger hormone," ghrelin has numerous functions in addition to telling your brain you're hungry. For example, ghrelin:

• Increases food intake and helps your body store fat.

• Helps trigger your pituitary gland to release growth hormones.

• Plays a role in controlling sugars and how your body releases insulin, the hormone responsible for processing sugar.

• Has a role in protecting your muscles from weakness and bone formation and metabolism

What is the difference between ghrelin and leptin?

Ghrelin and leptin are two of many hormones that control your appetite and fullness. They're involved in the vast network of pathways that regulate your body weight. Leptin decreases your appetite, while ghrelin increases it.

Ghrelin is made in your stomach and signals your brain when you're hungry. Your fat cells produce leptin. Leptin lets your brain know when you have enough energy stored and feel "full."

Ghrelin plays a role in the short-term control of appetite while leptin controls long-term weight control.

What does the ghrelin hormone do?

Ghrelin has several key functions. The hormone:

• Signals part of your brain called the hypothalamus to increase appetite.

• Promotes fat storage.

• Stimulates your pituitary gland to release growth hormones.

• Stimulates your digestive system to move food from your stomach through your small and large intestines.

• Contributes to controlling insulin release.

• Plays a role in protecting your cardiovascular health.

What triggers ghrelin?

Your stomach releases ghrelin when it's empty or mostly empty. Ghrelin levels are typically highest right before mealtimes.

Imbalance between these hormones is the major pathogenic mechanism involved in Obesity.

CHAPTER 2

CLINICAL CONSEQUENCES OF OBESITY / METABOLIC CHANGES

Your metabolism is the method involved with changing calories into energy completely to fuel your body's capabilities. At the point when your body has a larger number of calories than it can utilize, it changes over the additional calories into lipids and stores them in your fat tissue (muscle versus fat). At the point when you run out of tissue to store lipids in, the fat cells themselves become amplified. Expanded fat cells discharge chemicals and different synthetic compounds that produce an incendiary reaction.

Ongoing aggravation has numerous unfriendly well-being impacts. One way that it influences your digestion is by adding to insulin opposition. This implies your body can never again utilize insulin to proficiently bring down blood glucose and blood lipid levels (sugars and fats in your blood). High glucose and blood lipids (cholesterol and fatty substances) likewise add to hypertension.

Together, these joined gambling factors are known as metabolic disorders. They are gathered because they will generally build up one another. They additionally support further weight gain and make it harder to get thinner and support weight reduction. Metabolic condition is a typical calculated weight and adds to many related infections, including:

1. Type 2 diabetes. Stoutness explicitly raises the gamble of Type 2 diabetes seven-overlay in individuals appointed male upon entering the world and 12-crease in individuals allotted female upon entering the world. The gamble increments by 20% for each extra point you gain on the BMI scale. It additionally reduces weight reduction.

Cardiovascular sicknesses. Hypertension, elevated cholesterol, high glucose and irritation are all hazard factors for cardiovascular illnesses, including coronary corridor sickness, congestive cardiovascular breakdown, respiratory failure and stroke. These dangers increment connected at the hip with your BMI. Cardiovascular illness is the main source of preventable demise overall and in the U.S.

2. Fatty liver Disease. An abundance of fats circling in your blood advance toward your liver, which is answerable for sifting your blood. At the point when your liver starts putting away an overabundance of fat, it can prompt persistent liver irritation (hepatitis) and long haul liver harm (cirrhosis).

3. Kidney Disease. Hypertension, diabetes and liver sickness are among the most widely recognized supporters of ongoing kidney illness.

4. Gallstones. Higher blood cholesterol levels can make cholesterol amass in your gallbladder, prompting cholesterol gallstones and potential gallbladder illnesses.

Direct impacts

Abundance muscle to fat ratio can swarm the organs of your respiratory framework and put pressure and burden on your outer muscle framework. This adds to:

Asthma.

Sleep apnea.

Stoutness hypoventilation condition.

Osteoarthritis.

Back Paint.

Gout.

As per the U.S. Places for Infectious Prevention and Avoidance, 1 of every 3 grown-ups with stoutness additionally has joint pain. Reads up have shown that for each 5 kg in weight gain, your gamble of knee joint pain increments by 36%. Fortunately, along with working out, a weight reduction of 10% can altogether diminish joint inflammation-related torment and work on your satisfaction.

Indirect impacts
Stoutness is additionally related in a roundabout way with:

Memory and cognizance, including an uplifted gamble of Alzheimer's illness and dementia. Female barrenness and pregnancy complexities.

Discouragement and state of mind problems.

Certain tumours, including oesophagal, pancreatic, colorectal, bosom, uterine and ovarian.

CHAPTER 3

CAUSES OF OBESITY

Basically, obesity results from consuming more calories than your body can use. Many factors contribute to this. Some factors are unique to you. Some are embedded in our social fabric at the national, local and family level. In a sense, preventing obesity requires consciously addressing these multiple factors. Factors that increase calorie expenditure include:

• Ready-to-cook meals. In communities and households where highly processed fast food and instant meals are a staple, it's easy to consume a lot of calories. These foods are high in sugar and fat and low in fiber and other nutrients, which can leave you feeling hungry. Its ingredients promote addictive eating habits. In some areas, only these types of food are readily available due to cost and availability issues. The Centers for Disease Control and Prevention estimates that

40% of American homes live more than a mile from a health food store.

• Sugar is in everything. The food industry was not designed to keep us healthy. It's designed to sell products that inspire us and make us want to buy more. At the top of this list of products are sweets and sugary drinks with no nutritional value and lots of extra calories. But standard foods also contain high levels of sugar, making them more appealing and addictive. It's common enough to alter our taste expectations.

• Marketing and advertising. Extensive advertising promotes the products we need most, such as processed foods, candy, and sugary drinks, but the products the industry wants to buy the most. Advertising makes it seem like these products are a normal and necessary part of everyday life. Advertising also plays a big role in the sale of alcohol, which contains many empty calories.

• Psychological factors. Boredom, loneliness, anxiety and depression are prevalent in modern society and can lead to overeating. In particular, you may start eating certain types of foods that activate the pleasure centers in your brain—foods that tend to be high in calories. Eating to feel good is a basic human instinct. We evolved to find food, but that evolution has not kept up with the abundance of food that Western societies enjoy today.

• Hormones. Hormones regulate our hunger and satiety signals. Many things can disrupt these regulatory processes, from common things like stress and lack of sleep to less common things like genetic mutations. Hormones make you crave more food even when you don't need calories anymore. They can make it difficult to determine when you've had enough.

• Certain medications. Medications taken to treat other medical conditions can contribute to weight gain. These include antidepressants, steroids, antiseizure medications, diabetes medications and beta blockers.

Factors that reduce calorie consumption include:

I. Screen culture. As we work, shop, and socialize more and more online, we spend more and more time in front of our phones and computers. Streaming media and binge watching make it easy to sit and enjoy hours.

II. Employee changes. With the shift to automation and computers in the industry, more people are working at desks rather than standing. They can also work longer.

III. Malaise. Lack of exercise can snowball. Studies show that the longer you sit still, the more tired you are and the less motivated you are. Sitting stiffens, causes pain, and restricts movement. It also causes systemic stress and increases fatigue.

IV. Neighborhood design. Many people lack local places to be active, either due to access or safety issues. More than half of Americans don't live within half a mile of a park. They may not live in walkable neighborhoods, and they may not see others in their communities being active in day-to-day life. When there is no public transportation option, most people can only travel by car.

V. Childcare trends. Children spend less time playing outside than they used to. They spend more time in enclosed childcare environments, which may not have adequate space or facilities for physical activity. This is partly due to cultural trends that don't find it safe for children to play outside unattended. It's also due to inadequate access to public spaces and inadequate access to quality childcare. Many childcare environments substitute TV for free play.

VI. Disability. Adults and children with physical and learning disabilities are most at risk for obesity. Physical limitations and lack of adequate specialized education and resources can contribute.

Section 2: THE CURE

Treatment and Management

CHAPTER 4

LIFESTYLE MODIFICATION

Lifestyle modification is changing long-standing routines, usually related to eating or exercising, and keeping up the new behavior for weeks, months, or even years. Obesity is one of several diseases that may be treated with lifestyle change.

These includes

1. Dietary Changes
2. Changes in Way of life
3. Physical Activity
4. Behavioral therapies

DIETARY CHANGES

1.Dietary changes

You will have to adjust your diet specifically for yourself in order to lose weight. Cutting back on portions or between-meal snacking may be beneficial for some people. Others might find that adjusting what they eat rather than how much is more important. Increased plant consumption is advantageous for almost everyone. Fruits, vegetables, whole grains, and legumes typically contain more fiber and micronutrients while having lower fat content. They are more nutritious and can increase your feelings of fullness and satisfaction even when you consume less calories.

Diets that work.
There are tons of diet plans floating around the internet with hefty promises of quick weight loss. Of these diet plans, the ones that work the best are the plans that reduce the number of calories you eat and are easy to stick to over time.

The simplest diet approach is to increase your intake of vegetables, fruits, whole grains, and lean proteins, while avoiding sugary snacks and processed foods.

Diet plans, like the ones outlined below, can also be effective if they're done right. But you might need to do some trial and error before you find one that works well for you.

Counting calories

You must consume fewer calories than you expend in order to lose weight. Therefore, tracking your calorie intake is the simplest way to lose weight.

According to a 2014 peer-reviewed study, weight reduction regimens that include calorie tracking frequently result in greater weight loss than those that don't. Reliable Source.

Finding out how many calories you need to consume daily in order to lose weight is the first step. You may calculate this using calculators that are accessible online, such as this one. To find out how many calories you need, enter your current height, weight, gender, and level of exercise.

The next step is to record how many calories are present in each meal you consume.

This takes a bit of effort, but there are many apps and websites available to simplify the process.

Some of the most popular free calorie-counting apps or websites include:

• My Fitness Pal

• Lose It!

• FatSecret

Enter in the type of food you're eating and how much of it you ate. The app or website will do the rest. To make sure you're counting calories accurately, you may want to invest in a food scale.

Low-carbohydrate diets

A low-carb diet, such as the Atkins diet, the South Beach diet, or the ketogenic (or "keto") diet, entails consuming less carbs each day while consuming more protein.

These diets frequently limit daily carbohydrate intake to only 20 to 50 grams. When you consume this little carbohydrates, your body starts converting fat into ketones. Your body starts relying mostly on ketones for energy.

A high-protein diet, which has been found to burn more calories during digestion than carbohydrates or fat and helps keep you fuller longer, is encouraged by a low-carb diet.

According to one research, low-carb diets like the Atkins diet are more effective in helping people lose weight than other diet plans.

Vegetarian diets

Vegan or plant-based diets place a strong focus on consuming only complete foods, such as fresh produce, whole grains, and legumes, while eliminating processed foods, dairy products, and meat.

In one study with 75 overweight or obese patients, those who followed a vegan diet had substantial reductions in body weight, fat mass, and insulin resistance indicators.

A plant-based diet may also lower your chances of developing heart disease and other diseases.

Alternate-day fasting

By alternately fasting and eating, intermittent fasting is a technique for controlling calorie intake. When you fast, your insulin levels drop but your growth hormone levels sharply rise.

You may do this to preserve your muscle mass while losing fat. According to a 2018 comprehensive review and meta-analysis, this style of eating pattern can result in a 4 to 8 percentTrusted Source weight loss on average.

There are several ways to fast intermittently, including:

• The 5:2 diet, or alternate-day fasting.Five days a week you eat normally, and two days a week you limit your calorie consumption to 500 to 600.

• 16/8 technique.You can only eat for eight hours using this technique. For instance, you are only permitted to eat between 12 and 8 o'clock. After that, you observe a 16-hour fast.

Eat, Stop, and Eat.One or two times every week, you fast for 24 hours using this technique. For instance, you skip meals from supper the day before till dinner the next day.

2. Change in way of life

It takes much more than just nutrition to manage obesity. A change in lifestyle is also necessary. The adjustments do not have to be implemented all at once, though.

The following lifestyle modifications can be gradually incorporated into your regular routine:

• store fruits, vegetables, and wholesome snacks in your refrigerator.

Increase your water consumption.

• use a smaller plate.

• Consume food gently.

• refrain from eating when watching television.

• Be careful you get adequate sleep.

• park a distance from a building's door so you have to walk a distance to get inside

The escalator rather than the stairs

• Keep away from fast food outlets

• Consume meals high in fiber

• lessen your level of tension

• eliminate all sugary drinks; if you're having a hard time giving up soda, switch to diet soda or try sparkling water

• start your day with a healthy, high-protein breakfast, like eggs instead of cereal or bagels

• when dining out, ask for a take-home box and put half of your dish in it to eat the next day

• read food labels carefully and pay attention to what's considered a serving size and the number of calories in each serving

Making just a few of these changes can have a massive effect on your weight and overall health

• Cut out all sugary beverages; if you find it difficult to give up soda, try sparkling water or diet soda.

• Instead of cereal or bagels, start the day with a nutritious, high-protein breakfast like eggs.

• When eating out, request a take-home box, then portion out half of your meal to save for the following day.

• carefully read food labels, paying close attention to portion sizes and calorie counts for each dish.

Even a small number of these adjustments can have a significant impact on your weight and general health.

3. Increased Physical Activity

Diet and exercise are both essential for weight reduction and maintenance, as is common knowledge. Exercise, though, need not include a gym membership. One of the best forms of exercise for losing weight is just walking at a slow speed. Healthcare professionals recommend exercising for just 30 minutes each day, five days per week. A regular stroll before or after work, at lunch, or any other time might be quite beneficial.

Workout routines

A healthy lifestyle must include exercise. Physical and mental health are both improved by exercise. Moreover, it can aid in weight loss. To achieve your fitness goals, combine weight training with cardiovascular activity.

Aim to do cardio for no more than 30 minutes each day to start, and then increase it as needed.

Some ways to get cardio exercise include:

• jogging

• cycling

• power walking

• hiking

• swimming

Loss of muscle mass is common during dieting. To combat muscle loss, try lifting weights or doing body-weight exercises like pushups and situps at least twice a week.

Working out as an overweight person may be challenging for a beginner. However, it is essential to make a smooth transition and make working out as easy as possible. If you are obese, your weight might add more pressure and strain to your bones, joints, and muscles. Hence, it is integral to follow a workout routine that does not hinder the health of your body internally.

If you are overweight, various mistakes while exercising can do more harm than good. It is important to build flexibility as well as strength in your joints and muscles. In this article, we discuss some effective yet low-impact exercises you should follow if you are overweight to increase your joints' and muscles' strength as well as flexibility. This article discusses several low-impact workouts that you should do if you are overweight and want to lose weight.

Here are 7 simple low-impact workouts for beginners who are overweight:

I. Walk

Walking is arguably the finest physical exercise to include in your regimen if you are just starting out. Walking improves weight reduction and has a very modest impact. Additionally, it may improve lung function, blood circulation, and other bodily processes that might speed up weight loss.

II. Jog, not run.

Running could put stress on your joints and leg muscles if you don't gradually include it into your regimen. It's crucial to gradually build up your body's strength and suppleness. While still low-intensity, jogging can help you lose weight more quickly than walking.

III. A fixed cycle

Another excellent technique to build your body's flexibility and strength without putting it under stress is to use a stationary bike. Bicycling on stationary bikes is a healthier option because they may be stopped whenever it's convenient for the user.

IV. Adapted workouts

Modifying numerous well-known routines is a fantastic additional technique to make exercising simple and transitioning. For a novice who is overweight, exercises like push-ups, squats, leg lifts, etc. may be overly taxing or uncomfortable. Try modified low-impact variations of these exercises first, then gradually progress to the original forms.

V. Swim

If you are overweight, swimming is another excellent approach to reduce weight. Even while swimming seems low-intensity, it can really speed up weight loss. Swimming and water aerobics are great ways to lose weight as a beginner.

VI. Dance

Another enjoyable exercise you may include in your schedule as a beginning is dancing. Dancing is incredibly pleasurable and may be altered to the dancer's convenience. The release of happy hormones may be increased by dancing to beats and other rhythmic music, which could increase your energy levels even further.

VII. Yoga

Yoga may be customized to suit your needs, much like dance. Yoga is another low-intensity but high-impact exercise program that can speed up your weight loss. It has been demonstrated that yoga enhances the performance of several other bodily functions. This might hasten the process of losing weight even further.

In conclusion, balancing all the variables is the secret to healthy weight loss. It is best to ease into an exercise regimen as an overweight starter since pushing yourself too hard or overdoing it might leave you vulnerable to aches and accidents.Working exercise may be enjoyable and not taxing if you progressively increase your flexibility and strength. In addition, we advise you to consume a diet high in protein and other nutrients to provide your body the energy it needs for exercise.

4. Behavioral Therapies

Your weight reduction journey may be assisted by counseling, support groups, and techniques like cognitive behavioral therapy. Your brain may be rewired to encourage beneficial changes using these techniques. They can also assist you in controlling stress and addressing any emotional or psychological issues that might be hindering your progress. Having support on both the emotional and practical levels might be beneficial because weight and efforts to lose it influence us on many levels. Seeing a Metabolic Medicine Specialist might be helpful.

www.ingramcontent.com/pod-product-compliance
Lightning Source LLC
Chambersburg PA
CBHW071010260726

48661CB00007B/2882